Marathon Method

Essential Guide to Training for Your First Marathon

Selecting, training, and finishing
your first marathon the easy way

JOE DONOVAN

JULIANJOHN

Cover Design by Sean O'Connor
OhSeeDesign.com

Special Note: This edition of "Marathon Method, Essential Guide to Training for Your First Marathon" is designed to provide information and motivation to our readers. It is sold with the understanding, that the publisher is not engaged to render any type of medical, psychological, legal, or any other kind of professional advice. No warranties or guarantees are expressed or implied by the publisher's choice to include any of the content in this volume. Neither the publisher nor the author shall be liable for any physical, psychological, emotional, financial, or commercial damages, including, but not limited to special, incidental, consequential or other damages. Before beginning any fitness or training program, consult with a medical professional.

Printed in the United States of America

TABLE OF CONTENTS

Chapter	Title	Page

 Throughout this book, you'll see the TIP icon on the left many times. This book is filled with tips — the ones written in red next to this icon are those which I think are especially important. That said, I will now offer what I believe is the best advice I can provide: Before you start any exercise program, including training for a marathon, it is critical that you get a check up from your health care provider. I don't care if you are young or old, in shape or not, get yourself checked out to ensure you are healthy enough to run a marathon.

This is important!

PREFACE

The running of a marathon is a very special accomplishment. At 26.2 miles, the marathon distance seems vastly out of reach for even the most avid runners. In modern society, the finishing of a marathon signifies great dedication, physical stamina and mental toughness. It is a badge of honor bestowed upon those who cross the finish line.

But more than something to brag about, the marathon represents the completion of a wonderful, but very personal, journey. While no one runs a marathon alone, the life stories that accompany runners through their 26 miles run are unique to each runner.

For many runners, the running of a marathon comes after a retirement, the birth of a child, the loss of a loved one or the changing of an era. In other words, it was sparked from a life-changing event. For others, it signifies the beginning of a new, healthy lifestyle, replacing former bad habits with newer, more positive ones. But for all runners, the marathon is a race of hope. With the challenge, comes hope that in finishing a marathon, the runner's life will forever be positively changed.

This book will prepare you mentally and physically for the challenge and help you condition and train for your first marathon. Getting across the finish line requires more than hope, but it can't be done without it. This guide will give you the tools and information you need to achieve your goal—crossing that finish line.

This book is built on a simple theme, one that is easy to understand, yet difficult to believe.

You <u>can</u> run a marathon.

Yes, <u>*you*</u> can run a *marathon*.

I come to this assertion without ever having the good fortune of meeting you or knowing anything about you. I have come to understand this after having run with and coaching hundreds and thousands of people of all shapes, sizes, ages, and athletic abilities. It is with that knowledge that I can say that if you are healthy enough to run, (please, get a checkup), you <u>can</u> run a marathon.

Believe me when I say this. I believe it.

There are many books on the market that explain how to train for a marathon. This book is no exception; however, it does offer more. In this book I explain how to get started with your running, how to purchase gear, how to select a marathon, how to train for and otherwise prepare for a marathon, even including what to eat. I also explain what to expect before, during and after your race, as well as how to stay healthy during the whole process.

What makes this book different, and what makes me so proud of it, is that it covers a topic that every other book on the market neglects: the emotional, spiritual and mental aspects of the marathon.

While I believe that anyone can run a marathon, relatively few people actually decide to do it. But those who do, find the journey well worth their time, effort and dedication. For me and the people I've met on my marathon journey, it was one of the best things I ever could have done.

If you believe you can run a marathon, something I hope I convinced you of a few minutes ago, and you really want to accomplish your marathon goal, I'll get you to the finish line.

Stick with me, it s a great journey.

1: INTRODUCTION

> *"The running of a marathon is proof that ordinary people — people with jobs, families and worries — can do something extraordinary."*
>
> - Author unknown

I was almost there.

The parade of runners stretched like a conga line through the streets of New York. As the crowd clapped and friends and loved ones of runners waved signs of encouragement, I basked in my own glory.

I was going to finish a marathon.

I wasn't near the front of the pack — in fact, by the time I approached the finish line, the winners had probably already showered and enjoyed a decent meal — but I certainly wasn't near the end, either. My marathon finish put me right in the middle of the pack, and I couldn't have been happier.

As I turned right, near the famous statue of Christopher Columbus in Columbus Circle, I passed the 26-mile mark and took in the cool autumn air and the noise from the enthusiastic crowd. A tremendous feeling of pride and accomplishment swept over me as I neared the finish line. I felt terrific. In fact, I felt like I could run forever.

As the line of runners turned into Central Park, where the finish line would soon greet us, the scene seemed strangely familiar.

Like most of my fellow runners, my goal to run a marathon was set long ago. I was introduced to the marathon as a kid when the New York City marathon was featured on a Sunday morning sports show. I recall it as if it were yesterday. My brothers and I were crowded around the console TV, marveling at an aerial view of the starting line, which was being taped from a helicopter camera flying high above the towering Verrazano-Narrows Bridge. I was transfixed.

"Twenty-six miles?" I asked my older brother. "These people are going to run 26 miles?" The nearest McDonald's to our home was almost 26 miles away, so I was keenly aware of the distance. It seemed like a long way to travel, even by car.

I wanted to watch every minute of it, but was cut short by my mother's pleas for us to eat breakfast and, later, to join her and Dad for Sunday mass. After we returned from church, I resumed my place along with my brothers in front of the TV. We watched in awe as the winning runner sprinted toward the finish line, breaking the white tape as he raised his arms in victory. Soon after, streams of runners followed. Although the tape had long been broken, many of the runners raised their hands to the sky in celebration of their own individual victories.

"I could never run 26 miles," I told my brother. He paused a moment, not taking his eyes off the TV. We watched the runners on the screen—people of all shapes, sizes and ages—crossing the finish line. "You'd be surprised what you can do once you set your mind to it," he said.

I decided then and there that I, too, would run a marathon.

Some 19 years later, I ran up the small Central Park hill that hid the finish line. Just as I remembered from that Sunday so long ago, the road was framed on either side by grandstands, and I could hear an announcer's voice over a loud speaker as the crowd cheered. I tried to soak in the excitement of the moment and the pride I felt in myself.

As I ran, I thought of my friends, family and my fiancée, Leah, whose support meant so much to me over the months. I thought of my parents back in rural Wisconsin, who were watching live coverage of the marathon in the same room where I was inspired so long ago.

I also thought of my brothers and that Sunday morning after church. As I ran, my eyes welled with tears. I repeated to myself over and over, as if I couldn't believe what I had done, "I did it! I did it!"

That day, along with my wedding day and the births of my three children, was one of the best days of my life. Just as I couldn't know when my children were born the joy they would bring me, their father, when I crossed the finish line, I also could not comprehend the positive impact that marathon would have on the rest of my life.

Prior to running the marathon, I was an overweight and overworked office worker. Before I ran the marathon, I satisfied my desire to take on challenges by promising myself that *someday* I would do them. Prior to the marathon, I *let* things happen to me, instead of *making* things happen.

Through the marathon, I learned that I am in charge of my own destiny and that life is too short to put off my goals. Since that race, I've received my master's degree and am continuing to work toward my doctorate. I became a husband and a father, and I started a business. I have also run three more marathons and continue a cycle of running a marathon every other year. I'm proud to say that I have also competed in other endurance races, including a triathlon and a long-distance mountain bike race. As a result of meeting my goal and of accomplishing something as big as finishing a marathon, I gained the confidence in my own abilities to take charge of my life.

I did it, and I know you can, too.

I am of the belief that *anyone* with the proper health, time and desire can run a marathon. Over the years, I have been passed by people at mile 25 who weigh well over 300 pounds. I have run next to people in their 90's and was given words of encouragement on a difficult climb from a man who ran on artificial legs.

The marathon is for everyone. If you want to run a marathon, you can do it.

This is a book about running your first marathon. It is a *how-to* book, or at least part of it is. In it, I explain how to select and enter your first marathon, and I also provide information about gear and nutrition and how to care for your body. I also introduce you to some effective *mind game* techniques I have used over the years, along with many other helpful tips and techniques. You'll also receive my week-by-week training schedule — the same one I have used for four marathons.

In reading this book, I hope you benefit from more than just the *how-to's*. I hope to inspire you by explaining the awesome impact the marathon will have on the rest of your life. If you are like me, your first marathon is more than a race; it's a mission. I want you to accomplish your goal, and I want you to know that I'm with you every step of the way.

Happy running,

Joe Donovan

2: CONSIDERING THE MARATHON

> *"Anybody can do just about anything with himself that he really wants to and makes his mind to do. We are capable of greater than we realize."*
>
> - Norman Vincent Peale, author

A marathon? Who, me?

Each year more than half-million people run a marathon. Of that half-million, approximately 40 percent are first-timers. In some of the largest marathons in this country, the number of people running their first marathon often surpasses veteran marathoners by more than 2-to-1.

Many, many people have a secret goal of running a marathon. For some people, a desire to get fit has motivated them to strap on running shoes and start logging miles. For others, including myself, the marathon is a back-of-the-mind goal, something to accomplish "when the time is right."

In conducting research for this book, I talked with a lot of runners about their first marathon, and the issue of the "time being right" is one that comes up again and again. It seems that, for many new marathoners, a life-changing event got them to finally sign up and start training. I can't tell you how many people I have met who beat cancer and decided to celebrate with a marathon. What a wonderful and triumphant way to defeat a life-threatening illness!

For others, the birth of a child, the graduation of a child, the death of a loved one, a divorce or a marriage encouraged them to accomplish their marathon goal.

For some people, and I put myself in this category, there is a desire to make a healthy lifestyle change. Prior to my first marathon, I was an overweight and overworked aide to a U.S. Senator. I was getting married soon, and my fiancée and I wanted to have children soon after. I felt the time was right to make good on the promise I made to myself. I didn't know at the time I started my training that my completion of a marathon would have such a positive impact on my life — physically, emotionally and spiritually — and that I should have done it earlier. It is with that knowledge I offer this advice: If you want to run a marathon and have the time, the health and the wherewithal to do it, do it now. Don't wait for next year. Do it now.

The Marathon as a Commitment

As I said earlier, I believe any healthy person who has the desire and the time can complete a marathon. After all, running a marathon is simply completing a series of steps, each one bringing you closer to your goal. While the program I introduce you to in this book provides incremental steps that seem relatively easy, it is important for you to know that you cannot skip steps. You have to take each and every one.

Training for a marathon requires a lot of (surprise!) running. Running takes time. The amount of time will vary by week, but you should expect to spend between 45 minutes and one hour per weekday and several weekend hours training. Don't worry, we'll start slow and work ourselves up. The main point is to know that training does take time.

In addition, I have always noticed a need for more sleep when I'm training for a marathon. Either that or "I'm training for a marathon" is a great excuse and I end up sleeping more as a result. Either way, I require or want more sleep during my training periods.

Finally, training for a marathon is an added expense. As I will discuss in greater detail later, you don't need to spend a fortune on the best apparel and equipment, but there is a cost for extra shoes, clothing, entrance fees and travel expenses if your marathon is out-of-state.

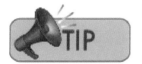 **Here's a Tip!** Training for a marathon takes time, and there are expenses. If you don't have the time to progress through the entire program or the extra cash for the right equipment, wait till you do.

Have a Heart-to-Heart Conversation with Loved Ones

Training for a marathon requires a personal commitment on your part. It also requires a commitment on the part of your partner or your spouse, your children and any other people who will be affected by your change in schedule and your training program.

It is important to discuss your marathon plans with these people before you decide you are going to complete your marathon. Be honest in explaining the time and the extra expense that will be involved.

It is also important that you to explain the reason(s) you want to run the marathon. (Guys, are you listening? This is important.) If running a marathon is a lifelong dream, like it was for me, explain it that way. Speak to the reasons why it is important for you. Make them understand why it is so important for you to do this so they can support and celebrate with you.

 **Here's a Tip!** It's quite likely that your partner or spouse will think your marathon idea is a little off the wall. Expect reactions from, "Are you nuts?" to "Are you sure you want to do this?" Give your partner/spouse some time to consider this commitment. Don't necessarily expect an immediate positive reaction.

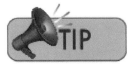 **Here's another Tip!** If you have kids, talk with them about this marathon. Use your marathon as a way to teach your children the importance of setting and reaching goals. Sit down with your children and discuss what the marathon means to you and what kind of commitment it will take, on your part and theirs.

So, you've had a check up, you have considered the time and expense involved in the marathon and you've talked with people who are close to you. Are you ready to take on your marathon mission? If so, let's discuss your first steps.

3: THE FIRST STEPS

> *"Running is the greatest metaphor for life,*
> *because you get out of it what you put into it."*
>
> - Oprah Winfrey, talk show host and marathon finisher

Congratulations. You've taken the first step on your marathon mission. This chapter provides information about your next steps. If you're anything like me, you will probably want to skip this section. Please don't. This section asks you to consider some important questions -- things that will help you down the road.

Let's begin with determining the time frame of your marathon.

Marathon Time Frame

Completing a marathon takes a lot of planning and preparation, and it is very important that you give yourself enough time to prepare for your marathon.

Some people who watch a marathon on TV or read the results in the newspaper set a goal to run that very marathon the next year. For most people, a year of training will allow them the time to establish a running base, lose a few pounds and complete an eighteen-week training program without a problem.

I am on a cycle of running a marathon every other year. For me, knowing that I am going to run a marathon on a particular day every other year means that I can officially begin my marathon training the day of the race in the year I don't run. For example, I knew I was going to run the New York City Marathon in 2007, so my official training kick-off was the day that marathon was run in 2006. I kept a calendar on my computer to mark off the days until the race.

Here again, a year for most runners will be enough time to train. But for others, completing a marathon will take more than a year. Talk with your health care provider and get their advice for your marathon time frame. Don't rush it. I have seen too many people fail to run their marathon because they try to accomplish too much in a short period of time.

As I mentioned earlier, training for a marathon requires successfully following many small steps. For many people, their first steps will be to lose weight, get active or get healthy. If you need to do this before you start your formal 18 to 20 week running program, no problem. Just give yourself plenty of time and keep on track.

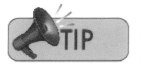 **Here's a Tip!** When you do decide what marathon to run, set an "official" start of your training. Put it on your calendar and do something special to recognize the date. I like to have a special, "Start of Marathon Training" run. When you set a start date, it's more difficult to postpone your training.

Selecting your Marathon

Yes, it is true that all marathons are the same distance, 26.2 miles (about 42.2 kilometers). While the distance is always the same, there is a great deal of differences between races.

Right from the start, it is important to note that the oldest and most famous marathon, the Boston Marathon, requires entrants to qualify in order to be accepted. That is, prior to running the Boston Marathon, you have to run another marathon, have a good time, qualify, and then enter Boston. Because of this, the Boston Marathon is not a beginner's marathon.

Speaking very generally, there are large, big city marathons and smaller, regional marathons. Here is a quick review.

Large marathons, like the New York City Marathon and the Chicago Marathon, attract between 30,000 and 40,000 runners from all over the world. These marathons are fun because you get to visit a new place from a unique perspective. If you love New York, there is no better place to see the five boroughs of the city than from the marathon course. Large marathons also have lots of added features, including lots of people along the course, usually well-stocked water stations, rest rooms, and on-course entertainment, like school bands and choirs.

I've run both the New York City and Chicago marathons and found both of them to be extremely organized and well-run. Due to the size and nature of the start, the New York City Marathon requires a little more forethought, but it is a wonderful first marathon. My experiences in Chicago were also good, though that race received a lot of negative attention in 2007 after the race was called off due to freakishly high temperatures. Despite this, I recommend either race for first-timers.

Keep in mind that some marathons, including the New York City Marathon, are so popular that not everyone is allowed to participate. This marathon uses a lottery to select entrants (something I will describe in detail later).

Other large races that have great reputations include the Los Angeles Marathon; the Marine Corps Marathon in Arlington, Virginia; the Seattle Marathon; the Paris Marathon; and the London Marathon.

Other smaller, but also well-known, marathons include: the Rock 'n' Roll Marathon in San Diego; the Steamboat Marathon in Steamboat Springs, Colorado; Grandma's Marathon in Duluth, Minnesota; and the Las Vegas Marathon.

There are dozens and dozens of smaller marathons all over the country. Smaller marathons are nice because they give runners lots of individual attention and tend to be less formal. These marathons often allow you to register right before the start and are often chosen because they are close by. This means you may be able to train on the actual marathon course.

I am a "large marathon" type of guy. I love the people, the noise and the big-city feel of larger marathons. However, I know lots and lots of people who prefer the smaller ones. The bottom line is to find a race that fits your expectations and go with it.

 **Here's a Tip!** There are dozens of marathons around the country. For a comprehensive schedule of marathons worldwide, go to www.MarathonGuide.com.

So, how should you select a marathon? Aside from the location of the marathon, there are some additional things that should be considered when selecting a marathon.

Is the course hilly? Unless your normal training takes you up and down lots of hills, I would avoid a hilly marathon as a first marathon. While many people do it, running a hilly marathon adds an extra layer of complication to an already challenging run.

Will it be held in the spring or fall? Marathons generally take place in either the spring or fall. While the actual temperature on marathon day for both a spring and a fall marathon will likely be similar, it is important to think of the type of weather you will experience in the weeks and months leading up to the race. If you live in a part of the country that has cold winters, keep in mind that a spring marathon will require you to put in your longest runs during the coldest times of the year. If you like the cold, no problem. If you hate running in the cold, you might want to consider a fall marathon when you can train in warmer weather.

I know a lot of people who love spring marathons. One of my neighbors, who is a marathon fanatic, loves to run during the coldest months. Not me. I hate running in the winter, and the cold Wisconsin winters keep me off the streets and on my treadmill. A spring marathon is simply not in the cards for me.

Another reason why I won't run a spring marathon, besides being a wimp, is because I believe it is important to run your race in conditions similar to those you trained in. That is virtually impossible in colder climates.

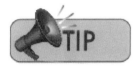 **Here's a Tip!** As I mentioned, the Boston Marathon requires that you qualify by running a prior marathon and finishing with a qualifying time. If you are bound and determined to qualify for Boston, check out the qualifying times on the Boston Marathon website, BostonMarathon.org, and make sure your first marathon is certified. You can learn more about this on the Boston Marathon website.

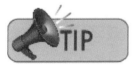 **Here's a Tip!** There are lots of things that must be considered when selecting a marathon, but I would like to make a strong pitch: Consider the possibility of traveling to a different city or part of the country to run your marathon. For me, part of the marathon adventure is being able to run in another city. My family and I look forward to flying to New York City or traveling to Chicago for my races, and my kids talk about it for months and months afterward. It makes the marathon even that much more special.

Registering for Your Marathon

Just about every marathon has its own website where you can find information about registering. Each marathon will have its own process, with some requiring you to register well in advance and others allowing you to register the day of the event. As I mentioned, some popular marathons, such as the New York City Marathon, require that you enter a lottery.

Whatever marathon you decide to run, review the process and register early. If you enter a marathon that uses a lottery, I encourage you to have a backup marathon that is run at roughly the same time. For example, I have the Chicago Marathon as a back-up in case I don't get in the New York City Marathon. Both marathons take place in the fall.

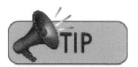 **Here's a Tip!** Some marathons, including the New York City Marathon, require entrants to be selected through a lottery. The good folks who run these marathons are usually pretty coy about your chances in the lottery, but I put it at about 30 percent. Want to know how you can get a guaranteed spot?

There are often two ways you can be guaranteed admission to a marathon. One is to run an earlier marathon really, really fast. Marathon organizers love to have really fast, Olympic-quality runners participate in their event because it lifts the stature of the marathon.

Since this is a book for first-time marathoners, I'm assuming you aren't training for the Olympics. This brings me to my second tip. In some cases, you can be guaranteed entry into the race if you agree to raise a specified amount of money for a participating charity. This is a great idea for you to help a worthy cause and get in the marathon of your choice.

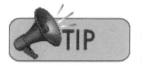 **Here's another Tip!** If you want to learn more about a particular marathon, you can always talk with someone who has already run it. Ask about the course, the crowd and whether there was enough water along the course and restrooms at the start and finish lines. Also, many race courses are shown on video at YouTube.com. Simply go to the site and search for the marathon. It's a cool way to see the course up close in a virtual format.

4: GEARING UP

"What spirit is so empty and blind, that it cannot recognize the fact that the foot is more noble than the shoe, and skin more beautiful than the garment with which it is clothed?"

- Michelangelo

One of the significant advantages of running marathons in this day and age is the dramatic improvements in shoes, running clothes and nutritional supplements. As you start on your marathon mission, make sure you have the right gear for the long road ahead. Let's take a look at the most important pieces of equipment.

Shoes

Not surprisingly, the most important single piece of gear is your shoes. Having good-fitting running shoes is critical, and trying to save a few bucks by scrimping on shoes is not a good idea.

Having said that, finding the right shoes for your feet is really difficult. There are so many different brands and models that it can be paralyzing. To get your head around finding the right shoes, it is important that you start with the right store.

Where do you go for help? Regardless of their size, most cities have a locally owned hole-in-the-wall running shoe store that is owned and employed by runners. This is where you want to buy your shoes. Not only will you get fitted properly in this kind of store, you will be taken care of by fellow runners who have been on their own marathon mission.

For the last 15 years, I have driven more than an hour to a small shoe store where the people measure my feet and expertly fit me with the perfect shoes. Sure, a pair of shoes at this tiny store costs a little more than if I went to the mall or purchased them online, but the service I receive is well worth the extra cost.

These stores are often hard to find. The best way to find the local runner's store is to ask fellow runners.

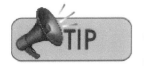 **Here's a Tip!** When you go to the store, you need to know that the right shoe for your foot might not be the best looking shoe in the store. In most cases, you can find a shoe that fits and meets modest demands for high fashion. But don't expect too much. Buy running shoes because they fit, not because they look good. Hey, we all want to look good. But do you want to know what is really ugly? Blisters. Enough said.

Socks

The second most important piece of gear, in my opinion, is your socks. When I first started long distance running, I wore basic white gym socks. What a mistake that was.

Regular old cotton gym socks are thicker than running socks and tend to hold onto moisture much more than a good pair of running socks. They are also much more likely to crease inside your shoe. Good running socks are lightweight, wick away moisture, and are much less likely to crease or have seams that cause blisters.

Blisters to long-distance runners are more than a pain — they can seriously wreck your marathon training. In most cases, blisters, especially serious blisters, can be avoided with good-fitting shoes and good socks.

I should point out that I think you will be surprised at the high cost of a pair of good socks. All I can say is that it's worth it and they tend to last a long time. You will thank me when you talk with a fellow runner who complains of blisters while you remain blister-free.

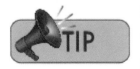 **Here's a Tip!** I like to wear the socks I'm going to wear in the race and in my training to the store when I buy my shoes. This ensures proper fit. I encourage you to do the same.

Two brands of socks that I highly recommend are WrightSock and SmartWool. Keep in mind that good socks cost a lot of money. The good news is they last a long time.

Support Items

According to some very bored researchers, the average middle-of-the-pack marathoner will take about 75,000 steps. Think about that. That is a lot of steps and a lot of bouncing.

It's hard to be subtle about this, so I'm just going to put it out there. Things bounce when you run — things that shouldn't bounce around, bounce around. Support is important.

A former high school athlete, I recall a poster that was hung in the boys' locker room admonishing us to wear proper fitting athletic supporters. The poster said failure to have the proper support would "result in irreversible damage." Now, I'm no health professional, but I do know that support is important.

So, when you are at the store, ask the sales person to show you different support gear. If you are a women and your salesperson is a man, don't be afraid to ask if there is a female salesperson who can show you a bra. They won't be offended, and you shouldn't be ashamed. Same thing goes for a guy. Talk with someone who uses the same stuff you'll wear.

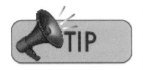 **Here's a Tip!** If it's uncomfortable in the store, it won't be comfortable when you run. Also, keep in mind you have to pay for comfort. Good-fitting support items are expensive.

Shorts, Shirts, Tights

As much as I can, I try to select the shorts and shirt I will wear for my marathon and wear then during my training. Sure, my neighbors might think I only own one set of running clothes, but what I give up in vanity, I make up for in knowing I won't have a problem with my clothing when I am at the starting line.

I learned this the hard way. A few years ago, I needed a new running shirt. My old one, which had served me through hundreds of runs and two marathons, was looking pretty shoddy. I went to my local running store and, with great care, selected and purchased a new shirt.

It seemed exactly like my old one — same manufacturer, same color, same size — so I tried it out on my next 20-mile run. Big mistake. While this shirt looked and felt exactly like my old one, the manufacturer had recently started treating the fabric with a new chemical that made the shirt reflective. It also made it very hot, especially around the 18th mile. The lesson: Find clothes that work and stick with them.

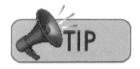 **Here's a Tip!** When you purchase shirts and shorts, take care to ensure the seams and tags are not going to cause problems. Getting back to the bounce factor, keep in mind that something as simple as a tag or a ill-positioned seam bouncing on wet skin for four hours will wreak havoc. I have seen men with bloody backs because of a tag and I've personally had broken skin due to a poorly fitting shirt that seemed perfect for a long run.

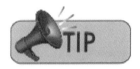 **Here is another Tip!** Keep in mind that the weather can change during your longer training runs and also during the marathon itself. Whenever possible, dress in layers that you can add or shed as the temperature warms up and cools down. I tend to run late and like to tie a long-sleeved running shirt around my waist that I can throw on if I get cold.

Hats, Watches, Sunglasses

I tend to do a lot of my longer runs along a paved trail that has become a favorite training place for other marathon runners. As a result, I tend to run with lots of other people who are training for marathons. One of the mind games (I'll explain mind games in greater detail later) I use is to count the number of runners who are wearing hats. During my last nine years of running, I have noticed more and more people, especially women, wearing visors and hats.

I'm not a hat guy myself, but many people swear by them to keep themselves cool and to keep the sun off their faces. I also see a lot of people wearing sunglasses and watches. Here again, I don't run with either, but a lot of people do.

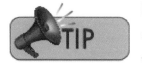 **Here is a Tip!** If you do wear a hat, sunglasses, a watch, a cape—whatever you wear—don't wait until you begin longer runs to start wearing it. Also, and I'll repeat this again later, if you wear a hat to train, wear it during the race. Find what works and stick with it.

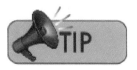 **Here is another Tip!** As I mentioned, I tend to do a lot of my running in the early morning and at night. Because my runs require that I cross a lot of city streets, I am always concerned about cars seeing me. Reflective gear helps, but I've found a better way to be seen. When I run, I carry in my hand a little LED light. It's made for putting on a bike, but because it is very small, it's easy to carry. It is also extremely bright and can be set so it blinks. As I run, I carry it in my hand so it is facing traffic. That way I make sure drivers see me. This is especially helpful when crossing dark intersections.

5: GETTING YOUR MIND AROUND YOUR MISSION

> *"Make your life a mission — not an intermission."*
> - Arnold Glasgow

Now that you have selected a marathon, signed up for it, been accepted and started training, it is time for you to take the next big step: getting your mind around your marathon mission. Training for a marathon requires a metamorphosis of sorts, taking you from who you are now into a marathoner. This section discusses training for your mind.

Sharing your Goal

I am often asked by first-time marathoners for advice. I always tell them the most important thing they can do is to tell as many people as they can (without being obnoxious) that they are training for a marathon. This step is important because it forces you to talk about your marathon with lots of people. This will not only keeps you focused, but it also means you can't back out. You made a goal, and you are going to accomplish it! In addition, talking about your marathon and sharing stories about your goal and your training turns you into a marathoner.

Some people think they turn into a marathoner the moment they cross the finish line. I disagree. I think a person turns into a marathoner when they believe they <u>can</u> cross the finish line. That is a subtle, but important, difference. Talking about your marathon puts you in a marathoner's state of mind.

If you are at all like me, when I ran my first marathon, I didn't look like a runner. I needed to shed a few pounds, I wasn't exactly light on my feet, and most people knew me as a suit-wearing office worker. I learned that a lot of people think marathoners have to be stick-thin running machines. I certainly didn't look the part, at least not in the eyes of friends and colleagues.

So, when I began telling people I was going to run a marathon, I got a lot of odd looks. In some cases, after I told a friend or colleague about my plans, they took a step back, looked at me from head to toe and said, "You? *You* are going to run a marathon?"

I have to tell you, I was a little stunned by this the first time it happened to me. But I felt better after talking with fellow runners who had this same experience. If it happens to you, don't feel bad, and don't let it keep you from accomplishing your goals.

The fact of the matter is the same people who initially reacted with surprise about my marathon mission became some of my most important supporters. It's not that they didn't believe in me, but rather that they were shocked and surprised at first to hear that I, someone who they would least expect, was announcing that I was going to run a marathon.

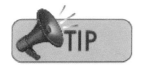 **Here's a Tip!** While you can run a marathon and not tell anyone about it, I think half the fun, especially for your first marathon, is in sharing your goal with other people. Be an inspiration to others.

Not only does this give you something to talk about, but I gained so much support from all kinds of friends and colleagues. One of my work colleagues, an older Catholic woman, asked me what time I did my long runs on the weekends. She said she wanted to know so she could pray for me at the exact moment when I needed the most help. To me, that was a wonderful gesture.

Another colleague, a runner herself, put a different marathon quote on my office door every week to keep me inspired. Yet another friend took me to lunch every Friday, making sure I ate a big bowl of pasta so I would have the requisite fuel for my long Saturday runs. One Friday, I suggested soup, to which he adamantly refused, informing me that our Friday pasta lunch was his role in my training. It was his job, and he was taking his role quite seriously.

The bottom line is to do yourself a favor and tell people about your goals — just don't get too disappointed if their reaction is different than what you expected.

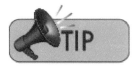 **Here's a Tip!** You will receive lots of positive comments from friends about your marathon plans. Take mental stock of these comments. I encourage you to keep a running list of people who share your excitement about the race, people you can call for encouragement and to share the good news with when you finish.

You are a Machine

When I ran my first marathon, one thing that I found interesting was how much better it made me understand my own body. Because you are forcing your body to do something you have never done before, namely logging lots and lots of running miles, you will become aware of all of the little aches and pains that come with the training. But you will also become aware that your body is a machine.

We all know that we are supposed to give our body proper nutrition and plenty of rest. We learned that in elementary school, right? Well, training for a marathon will make you experience the downside of eating the wrong foods and in failing to get enough sleep. A long night of beer and onion rings before a long run simply won't work. Relying on your body to get you through those long runs will force you to make sure you put the right fuel in your tank and that you are getting enough sleep. That was a true wake-up call for me, and a lesson that has served me well since.

I think this step is one of the most positive ones you'll take in your marathon journey. I have seen lives change, almost overnight, as a result of people's change in perceptions about their bodies. I have seen people, who were significantly overweight and hooked on fast food, start packing a lunch, losing weight and keeping off those extra pounds. I have also seen people who have smoked most of their lives kick the habit once and for all.

These people knew that smoking and eating fast food wasn't consistent with their new lifestyle as a runner, and they dropped those bad habits and took on healthier ones.

Do you have any bad habits?

Self-Talk:

There are volumes of books written about the importance of self-talk and keeping a positive mental attitude. While there is a lot of information out there about this, I want to pass on three pieces of advice.

First, I want to offer some advice a college professor passed along to me a long time ago: Don't ever let negative talk enter your mind. Ever.

I'm sure you've heard the same thing before, but, like me, you probably didn't think too much about it. But when running a marathon, it is especially important that you stay positive and focus only on the positive, rather than dwelling on the negative.

Allow me to be a little more specific and blunt. When I ran my first marathon, I was overweight. I hadn't done that much running, I didn't have the best diet, and I wasn't exactly a picture of fitness.

Add to that the fact that I didn't know what I was doing and that 26 miles is a hell of a long way to run. If I had focused on all of that, I would have never run a marathon.

You see, running a marathon is a calculated gamble, where if you do the right preparation, your body and mind will carry you 26 miles. It is calculated leap of faith. This brings me to my second self-talk item: Don't be logical.

What's that, you ask? Look, if you are one who dissects everything in an attempt to be logical about every decision, I have some advice for you. Don't allow yourself to think logically about your marathon. That's because there is almost nothing logical about the marathon, at least when you are training and running your first one. So, don't try to justify the logic. You have to be disciplined in not allowing yourself to think about why you *can't* do it and only think about why you *will* do it. Don't let negative self talk creep into your mind. And don't be logical.

Last, but not least, I want to talk about your becoming a marathoner. As I said earlier, I believe runners become marathoners not after they cross the marathon finish line, but when they first believe they can run the marathon. In this way, it is important that you start to view yourself as a marathoner. When you are out for your training runs, tell yourself you are on a very important, life-changing mission. You are doing something extraordinary: You are a marathoner!

Before moving on, I want to share something else with you. By this point in this book, you should be proud of what you have accomplished so far. You have decided to do something many people want to accomplish, but very few people actually do. Good job.

Now, let's get running.

6: GET RUNNING: CREATING YOUR BASE

"When you put yourself on the line in a race and expose yourself to the unknown, you learn things about yourself that are very exciting."

- Doris Brown Heritage,
five-time World Cross-Country Champion

Ask anyone who has ever run a marathon what the most difficult part of the process is and they'll likely tell you it's not the last mile, but the first one. As with any challenging, long-term goal, the most challenging step is getting started. This chapter will help you do just that.

I generally don't start chapters with tips, but I'm making an exception in this case. There is a 50 percent chance that what I am going to explain next is going to happen to you, so I want you to pay attention.

When most people decide to start running, they are excited about their first run. They lace up their new shoes, throw on their new running shorts, spend a lot of time warming up and stretching and enthusiastically make their way out the door for their first run. They expect a nice, easy run with the wind at their back and their heels kicking up dirt behind them. They are pumped up and so excited!

Guess what? That very first run isn't going to go well. As a matter of fact, it's going to go very badly. Bu the time you're about two blocks from your house, you're going to feel winded, your legs are going to feel like boat anchors, and the first thing that is going to go through your head is: I can't even run one mile, so how am I going to run 26 miles?

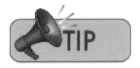 **So, here's your Tip!** Remember what I said about negative self-talk? Don't do it. You should know that your first run is going to be very bad. Don't worry. I don't care if you only go 100 feet. You will run a marathon. Don't defeat yourself.

The Pre-Program / Base-Building Phase

Often, when experienced runners talk about training for a marathon, they refer to the specific training program they follow. In that context, a marathon program is a 16-18 week program that prepares the runner for the marathon.

These programs are very specific and prescriptive. They are created to add miles at certain times and allow the runner to build strength and endurance. They also include time for rest prior to the big race. I include an 18-week training program later in this book.

But all these programs, including mine, require a baseline level of fitness prior to beginning. If you've been running three to five days per week (15 to 20 miles a week), and can comfortably run six miles and have been doing this for two months, you are ready to begin your training program. If not, you should adapt this pre-running program to work for you.

Creating a solid base for your training is very important, as it will ensure you are strong when you begin building miles on our training program. This base is like the foundation of a building — you need a strong base on which to build later.

Since I don't know your current fitness level, I'm going to assume it is pretty low. That is, I'm going to assume you are healthy enough for training (you did get that check-up, right?) but either you aren't running or you don't have a good base yet. The first thing we are going to do is to get you running. After that, we're going to establish a base of fitness before we get to the program. Keep in mind that for some people, this pre-program may be relatively short. For others, it will take longer.

Also keep in mind our goal at this stage is, again, to be able to run three to five days per week, for a grand total of between fifteen and twenty miles, and to be able to comfortably run six miles. (Did I just sense self doubt? You can do it. I promise.)

Getting Started

For the first couple weeks, or whenever you are comfortable to move on, I want you to do something I call the run-walk. The key is to run for a few minutes and to walk for a few minutes. I think it works best when you run slowly and walk briskly. Keep in mind that you will be pushing yourself and may get winded, but you should not feel any pain. If you do, talk with your health care pro.

Also, I want you to know that while our training program will be very prescriptive, this part of the program isn't. Do what works for you with the goal of getting to a point when you can run for 30 minutes straight.

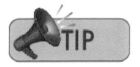 **Here's a Tip!** Stretch well. I find that most people have some knowledge of stretching and know that stretching is important. The problem is that most people simply don't do it. They should. Get in the habit of stretching each muscle group from your toes to your neck. In addition, stretching isn't something you should only do just before your run; it is also something you should do after your runs as part of your cool-down routine. As you will see, training for a marathon is largely a set of routines. Do yourself a favor and make gentle and slow stretching a part of your routine. See the chapter on stretching for more information.

Let's Get Started!

Week One

For the first week or so, simply run for one minute, then walk for five minutes and repeat the cycle three times. Do this three or four times a week for the first week. Remember to run s-l-o-w-l-y.

If that's too easy, run two minutes for every five you spend walking. For now, keep your walking to five minutes between each run. This will give you plenty of time to recuperate after each period of running.

Week Two

Once your one-minute runs become easy (hopefully in a week or so), bump it up to two minutes of running, then walk for five minutes, and repeat three times. Again, try to do this three or four times in a week.

How are you feeling? Are you stretching?

Week Three

All right, we are on a roll. When you are ready (again, hopefully within a week), let's bump it up to running for four minutes and walking for three, repeating three times. Keep that up for four run-walks per week.

Week Four

Looking good. We are well on our way. This week, you are going to run for six minutes, keeping your walking time to three minutes and repeating twice. If you are feeling strong, repeat for a third time for a total of eighteen minutes.

Week Five

Keep it up, you are doing great. This week, you will walk for two minutes and run for eight minutes. You will repeat this three times and do this four times a week.

Are you hanging in there? Feeling good? Remember, run slowly and stretch before and after your runs.

Week Six

Let's turn it up a notch. This time after you stretch, you will walk for two minutes before running for nine minutes. Repeat this three times. Get four good sessions in this week. I encourage you to take a nice, long walk over the weekend. Wear the clothes you wear when you run, including your shoes, and try to walk for at least forty-five minutes.

Week Seven

This is a big week. You will walk for one minute and run for twelve minutes. You will repeat this three times, and do four sessions during the week. Again, get a good walk in this weekend.

Week Eight

Congratulations on making it to week eight! For your first run this week, try walking for 5 minutes to begin and end the workout, and run for 20 minutes in between. By the end of the week, try to run for 30 minutes without stopping.

Aim to run for 30 minutes four times per week, and you'll notice your stamina and fitness will continue to improve.

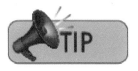 **Here's a Tip!** Use your breathing as your guide when running. You should be able to carry on a conversation while running, and your breathing shouldn't be heavy.

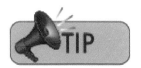 **Here is another Tip!** Drink water at the end of your workouts to rehydrate. If it's hot and humid, you should also drink some water (about 4-6 ounces) halfway through your workout.

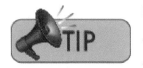 **Here's another Tip!** Now is a good time to join a local running club. Most large cities have a club that has training programs and classes for new runners. Not only are these clubs a great way to get started in running, but they are a great way to meet people.

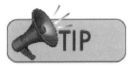 **Here's a Tip!** Take care in selecting who you run with. I'm not only talking about running with someone who runs the same distance and pace as you, but also someone you are very comfortable with. There are some rather unglamorous facets of long distance running. Burping and passing gas is sometimes inevitable, so make sure you are comfortable being seen at your worst in front of this person.

 **Here's a Tip!** Prior to running a marathon, I think it is a good idea to run some local road races. In most parts of the country, these races or "fun runs" are plentiful. Not only is this a great way for you to experience a marathon on a much smaller level, but you get used to the lineup, running in crowds, and taking water while you are running.

7: MIND GAMES

> *"People say I'm crazy.*
> *I've got diamonds on the soles of my shoes."*
> - Paul Simon, from the song
> "Diamonds on the Soles of Her Shoes"

An aspiring marathoner recently asked me, "What is the most important thing a new marathoner should know?" I didn't have to think, not even for a second. "The most important thing anyone preparing for their first marathon should know is that the marathon is 90 percent mental," I said.

I know this sounds cliché, but it's true. The requirement for successfully running a marathon are to avoid getting bored, paying attention to what your body is telling you, dealing with the aches and pains that will inevitably occur, and keeping a good mental attitude. The physical side is easy: You just have to get off the couch and run. It's the mental part that is the hardest.

This chapter provides tips to help keep your head in the game and train your mind as you train your body.

Don't Get Bored

An experienced runner once told me that he knew he was on his way to becoming a marathoner when his mind started wearing out before his body did. It didn't make much sense to me at the time, but as I got in better shape and my mileage went up, I started understanding.

You see, at a certain point, as your mileage increases, there is a tendency, especially for a new marathon runner, to get bored and, in some cases, feel a little lonely on their longer runs. In this way, a 20-mile run requires a lot of physical training, as well as a lot of mental preparation.

I'll admit when I ran my first marathon I hated the long runs. I hated them not because they were physically grueling — they weren't really. I hated them because I got bored. But over the years, I changed the way that I prepared for my long runs, and now I love them.

The key to not becoming bored is to stay focused on something. In the week prior to my long runs, I prepare by making a list of things I need to figure out during the week, things which I can give some serious thought to when I run. These can be mundane things, like should I get the black suit or the navy suit, or more serious, such as should I accept the promotion or start my own business.

One of the terrific byproducts of running a marathon is that I often make good choices because I can seriously consider the options. In this regard, the time you set aside for running can also be your most productive time.

I also use my running time to relax. During the week, I make a deal with myself not to worry about things. Instead, I allow myself to worry about whatever is bothering me during my run. For example, when I run, I'll worry about whether it is going to rain during an upcoming outdoor party I am hosting. Beyond prompting action, worrying for the sake of worrying isn't productive or beneficial, so I deal with it when I run. Specifically, I might allow myself to think about the presentation, but only for a mile or two. After that, I mentally try to leave it behind me as I run ahead. Try it. It works!

In addition to thinking, planning, and worrying, I spend a lot of time praying when I run. It's weird to write this because I am not the most spiritual person in the world. But there is something about the calming nature of running and the rhythmic sound of steps that allows me to think deeply about things that normally I don't or can't think much about.

So, after hating the time spent on longer runs, I learned to really love that time and look forward to it.

It Will Hurt, Sometimes

While I believe following the advice in this book will get you to the finish line, there is nothing I can do to help you with the fact that running a marathon can be a little painful. Based on my experiences, it is part of the process.

For example, on my longer runs, I can generally predict the time my legs will begin to ache, which is around mile seventeen. It's always minor, and the pain is more annoying than anything. But here again, it is important to recognize these pains without letting them sidetrack you.

Be smart about the pain you are feeling. If you have a very sharp pain or pain that either doesn't go away or leaves you with the feeling something just isn't right, see your health care professional. Don't mess around. If your pain is less serious, don't let it sidetrack you.

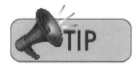 **Here's a Tip!** The way I deal with inevitable aches and pain while I am running is to welcome it. That's right. I force myself to think of the upcoming pain, like I am meeting up with an old friend who will run with me for a while. When I feel the aches beginning, I say to myself, "There you are old friend; how are you?" Then, I literally imagine myself running next to an old friend.

I know it seems strange. I felt that way when I heard this advice. But it works.

Do System Checks

If you get really good about thinking and praying when running, it's often easy to forget about making sure your body has what it needs to continue. With that in mind, I force myself to do a *quick systems* check at every mile-marker to see if I am hungry, need water or have an unusual pain. If you don't have a lot of experience running long distances, this may seem unnecessary, but it isn't. Believe me when I say it is very easy to lose track of what your body needs when you are lost in your thoughts during a long run.

Stay Sharp

You've probably heard of the "runner's high" before. It's the feeling of euphoria that comes from long, strenuous activity, such as running. While I don't know that I've felt high as a result of my running, I certainly feel better mentally, and often physically, after a nice long run. That is part of the reason I keep running!

What you probably have not heard of is what I describe as a "runner's fog." The fog I describe is the mental state of being where you are not actually thinking about running, yet you continue to run. It's similar to daydreaming.

Have you ever had to drive a long way over a period of a few days, and you lose yourself in your own thoughts? Then, all of a sudden, you realize that you've traveled a long way without even really remembering it? That's similar to runner's fog.

I tend to get "foggy" when I run the same course over and over again. Something about the familiarity of the course causes me to daydream. I've talked to some people who love the runner's fog because it helps them relax. While this is true, there is a downside to falling victim to the fog.

When I am less alert in my running, I often forget to do the things that are important—including taking in water and food. I also make dumb choices, like crossing streets without looking or tripping over things in the sidewalk.

In 2005, I was halfway through a long run and tripped on a small branch that had fallen on the sidewalk. I "came to" when I was sprawled across someone's yard, covered with mud and had a nasty scrape on my hand. The lesson here is to try to stay sharp. Keep your mind active. Stay relaxed but keep your head in the game.

Think About Staying Motivated

My guess is that if you talked with 100 people who have run marathons, you would get 100 different tips on staying motivated. I could give you lots of specific tips, but part of finding what works for you is coming up with your own motivation.

I will say this, however. I have young kids, and I get them involved in my training. If you haven't already noticed, I'm big into goal-setting. A few years ago, when we were on a family trip, my daughter, then five, asked how long 26 miles was.

To show her, I reset the tripometer. As 10, then 15, then 20 miles went by, she kept remarking, "Wow, that is a long way to run!" This led to a longer conversation about running. Her questions ran the gambit: "Do you ever get tired?" "Do you sweat?" "What do you think about when you run?" The questions went on and on. It was priceless.

Then, she asked a question that got me thinking. "Dad," she said. "What do the bottoms of your shoes look like after you run that far?"

I decided that for my next run, she and I would use a black permanent pen to draw a design on the bottoms of my shoes to see if there was any sign of the mark when I returned. Before my next long run, I turned over a shoe and asked her to make a design. She did. Then, I gave her a kiss and skipped out the door for my run.

Late in my run, I was smiling as I thought about the conversation and the design we drew. Thinking back, I recalled that her design looked like diamonds on the bottoms of my shoes. Instantly, an old Paul Simon song popped in my head. "People think I'm crazy; I've got diamonds on the soles of my shoes."

To this day, we draw diamonds on the soles of my shoes before my big runs. My kids get such a kick out of it; it's very motivating for me while I'm running. It's almost like they are running with me.

The bottom line here is that when it comes to motivation, no one can tell you what will work. You have to find your own motivation.

8: FEED THE MACHINE. AVOID THE WALL.

> *"The marathon is all about energy management."*
>
> - Frank Shorter, gold medalist in the marathon, 1972 Olympics

The Wall

By now, you've probably heard of "the wall" in the context of running a marathon. The concept of the wall was originally coined to describe what happens to many runners late in the marathon. "Hitting the wall" or "bonking" is when a runner experiences great muscle fatigue, making it very difficult to run. In some cases, hitting the wall also entails extreme dizziness, nausea and confusion.

I've hit the wall more than my fair share of times, and the best way I can explain it is to say that it feels like I'm pulling a Volkswagen as I run. I've talked with other runners about their experiences with the wall and everyone experiences it a little differently.

The first time I experienced the wall was at the end of my second 20-mile run before my first marathon. I ran especially early that morning and left my apartment, having eaten only half a bagel and a glass of juice. I typically didn't get hungry until later in the morning and didn't think it would matter much.

I was on mile 19 when I started feeling weird. I wasn't tired, but I felt dizzy and a warm sensation swept over my body, as if I had walked into a steam room. A few minutes later, it became clear something was wrong. I was nauseous and tired. I completed my run and took in some Gatorade. Within a few minutes, I started feeling better. While it was happening, it was both strange and scary.

So, what is the wall? To hit the wall is basically to run out of energy. A more exact explanation requires some science. Here goes...

The fuel that is used by runners is typically carbohydrates and fats. Carbohydrates are used by the body in the form of blood glucose and glycogen.

It is true that fats are also burned by the body in the form of fatty acids in the bloodstream and muscle triglycerides (molecules that contain fatty acids). It might seem like it would be best for your body to use up all of your body fat first, but it doesn't work that way. Burning fat requires a lot of oxygen circulating in your bloodstream, which is something your muscles also need for running. But your body can use carbohydrate fuel with or without oxygen, so our bodies use carbohydrate fuel first.

When we first begin running, about three-quarters of our energy comes from carbohydrates and the rest comes from fatty acids. However, as we progress in our long runs, we use up our carbohydrates and our bodies begin to burn more fatty acids. Here is the issue. Even if you load up on carbs, your muscles and your liver store only about 2,000 calories of carbohydrates that can be burned as fuel. That is only enough to get you to 18 or 20 miles.

After that energy has been burned, you hit the wall. At this point, your body starts burning fat. However, because you don't have a lot of extra oxygen to help metabolize the fat, this burning of fat is much less efficient and creates lactic acid as a by-product. The result, in unscientific terms, is you feel like your legs have turned into Jell-O. Not good.

The best advice I can give you about the wall is not to hit it. The bottom line is that with proper nutrition prior to, during and after your race, as well as listening to your body, you will never have to hit the wall.

In that context, let's talk about nutrition.

Nutrition for the Marathoner

Nutrition is one of the most important topics to consider in your marathon preparation. The best training schedule in the world is worthless if the fuel you expect your body to run on is junk. However, I know that the topic of nutrition can be confusing and overwhelming. My goal in discussing nutrition for the marathoner is to provide you with the basics.

The simple basics of marathon nutrition are that in order to be successful in your race, you must ensure that you remain well-hydrated and maintain an adequate supply of glucose. These are the two commandments of marathon nutrition, and if this is the only thing you take from this section, I've been successful.

There are, of course, other nutritional items you should consider. As we discussed earlier, your body is a machine that requires fuel. Without this fuel, it won't run. It's that easy. With this in mind, it is important you pay careful attention to the foods you put into your body. You probably won't be surprised when I urge you to make sure you have adequate vegetables and fruits. Also, ensure that you have plenty of protein in your diet. Personally, I'm not a big meat-eater, so I rely on eggs, beans, seafood and (if I'm really hungry) soy. Of course, make sure you have plenty of carbohydrates in your diet. Fruits and vegetables are a good source of carbs, as are whole grains.

I tend to stay away from processed carbohydrates, like white bread. Instead, I try to eat things like wheat bread, sweet potatoes and long grain rice.

Over the years, there has been a lot of debate about how many of your calories should come from carbohydrates. Based on many conversations and my own experience, my rule of thumb is that 65% of your calories should come from carbs. Finally, try to stay away from high-fat foods, food with a lot of empty calories (like soda and candy), and any fried foods.

Eating for the Long Run

Marathon rookies often ask me what they should eat before their long runs and before the race. Typically, they're asking if they should "carbo-load." Carbo-loading is just what it sounds like — eating extra portions of carbohydrates prior to a long run or race.

The answer is yes. I advise new marathoners to begin carbo-loading two days before their long run or race to make sure their muscles store as much glycogen as possible. In practice, this means adding an extra portion of carbohydrates to every meal in your otherwise balanced diet. In addition, take in an extra glass of water because as the body increases its glycogen stores, it also increases the amount of stored water.

Immediately prior to a long training run or the marathon itself, I make sure I am well-hydrated. I also eat a light, but high-carbohydrate, meal no later than two hours before the race or run. And, by all means, take advantage of the water, sports drinks and other glucose-containing foods offered at the aid stations!

Keep in mind that I prepare for my long runs (those in excess of 16 miles) in the same way I do my marathon. With that in mind, I try to eat the same way I will the day of the marathon and also try to replicate when and what I will drink. Then, when it comes to the day of the marathon, I know what works and my body will expect what I am providing it.

In the week before your big runs and during the marathon itself, make sure you are well-hydrated. You are also carbo-loading at this time, so drinking water is best. Research has shown carbohydrates convert to glycogen more effectively when accompanied with water.

As mentioned above, carbohydrate-loading begins three days before the marathon. Choose foods for lunch and dinner that are high in carbohydrates (e.g., pasta, potatoes, rice, etc.). However, don't neglect fruits, vegetables and some protein sources. Try to significantly scale back on fats during this time.

 **Here's a Tip!** If you are traveling by plane to your marathon destination, carry bottled water with you. Flying at high altitudes causes dehydration.

What the Gel?

One of the techniques that people use to ensure they keep enough fuel in the tank as they run is to use sports gels. The most popular gel, and the one I am familiar with, is Power Gel made by Power Bar. Another popular brand is Gu.

The gels are available in many different flavors, the most popular being chocolate. Imagine really, really sweet cake frosting, and you have a sense of the taste and consistency of the gels.

The gels are packaged in small 40 gram foil containers that fit in the palm of your hand. Each gel foil packs a walloping punch of carbohydrate calories that are easily absorbed by your system. There are many differences of opinion about using gels. It is important that you take the gels with water. If you don't have water, your body can't easily absorb the gel and you're likely to get sick.

I'm a big believer in gels and have for a long time urged new marathoners to use them. Generally, I tend to take one gel after my 10th mile and after my 20th mile, carrying them in my hand as I run.

In following up with some people to whom I've recommended gels, I've learned some runners can benefit from them, while others find them unnecessary or problematic in that the sweet mixture sours their stomach. Give them a try to see if they work for you.

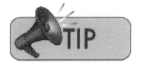 **Here's a Tip!** Once again, you should replicate what you've done in training when you are running your marathon. If you use gels for training, you should plan to use gels for your marathon.

Water or Sports Drinks

Another question I've received from many people over the years is: Should I drink water or sports drinks? Here is a simple rule of thumb: In most cases, water should be your drink of choice. You should drink lots of water during the day for your general health, and you should drink water for all your runs lasting under 90 minutes.

Sports drinks, such as Gatorade, should be consumed for runs lasting over 90 minutes. I find my stomach has a hard time late in the race drinking straight Gatorade, so I tend to mix water and the sports drink. During my training runs, I dilute Gatorade with water and put it in a water bottle. During the marathon itself, I take a cup of Gatorade and take two sips and take a cup of water and take two sips and dump the rest of both.

 **Here's a Tip!** It is very important that you develop a good routine of drinking fluids while you run. Don't rely on your thirst mechanism to indicate signs of dehydration because it is very difficult to "catch up" on your fluid requirements if you are already dehydrated. You have to keep your fluids up by taking in fluids on a regular basis while you run.

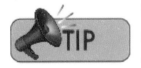 **Here's another Tip!** You may have heard news stories about people who drink too much water while they run and have other problems. Yes, you can drink too much while you run. Don't go nuts by drinking excessive amounts of water or sports drink while you run; just drink enough to maintain good fluid levels.

During the marathon, I drink two sips of water every mile and add two sips of sports drink every other mile. If it's hotter, I drink more.

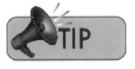 **Here's another Tip!** Speaking of sports drinks, find out what brand and flavor of sports drink will be distributed along the race course and use the exact kind and exact flavor when you train.

 **Here's another Tip!** Pay attention to the color of your urine. Generally, your urine should be clear with only a slightly yellow tint. Urine that is darker suggests you are dehydrated and need to drink more water.

9: AVOIDING INJURY / STRETCHING

> *He's going the distance.*
> *No trophies, no flowers, no flashbulbs, no wine.*
> *He's haunted by something he cannot define*
> *Bowel shaking earthquakes of doubt and remorse*
> *Assail him and impale him with*
> *monster truck force.*
>
> - The band Cake, from the song, "The Distance"

It is important to note upfront in this chapter, which is about injuries, that the single most important determinant of whether you will get injured has already been discussed. In my opinion, staying alert and in tune with your body is the single best way to avoid injury. In your training log, you should be making note of new aches and pains. Describe the pain in detail, along with its severity. Then, you and your trainer have a reference, where you can go back and determine when the injury started.

We also talked about proper fitting shoes and gear. Your body takes a tremendous amount of pounding in training runs. Finding the right shoes for your feet and running style will save your knees, and wearing good socks will keep blisters away.

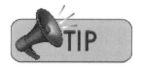 **Here's a Tip!** Don't underestimate the damage that blisters can cause. A severe blister, especially one that is infected, can keep you off your feet for weeks. Treat blisters immediately and do what you can to avoid getting them in the future.

There are two issues related to injuries that we have not yet discussed. The first is pain. As I noted earlier, you will have aches and minor pain, but when is a minor pain something to worry about? We'll discuss that next. We'll also discuss stretching.

Let's get started...

Pain

By this time in the book, you are probably tired of me telling you this, but I am compelled to say it once again: Make sure you see a health care professional before you begin training. I'm going to change my message slightly in this chapter and tell you that not only should you see your health care pro at the *beginning* of your training, but the two of you should stay in touch *during* your training. Remember earlier in this book when I said your body is a fine-tuned machine? Well, think of your health care professional as a mechanic.

The single best tip I can give you is to keep minor injuries from turning into major injuries. With the number of miles you are logging each week, you will have some minor aches and pains. But how can you, as a beginner marathoner, know whether an ache or pain is something to be worried about?

I can't tell you that. I can't tell you because I don't want to. I can't tell you because I don't know your body. Only your health care pro can tell you that.

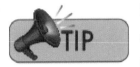 **Here's a Tip!** After you have your pre-training check up, make another "check in" appointment to talk about the aches and pains you know you will have. Schedule that appointment with your doctor, nurse practitioner, physician's assistant or with a trainer. More and more clinics now have trainers on staff. They are a terrific resource for you.

Stretching

Stretching and warming up your body prior to running is extremely important. Learn how to stretch every muscle group with long, slow stretches. Flexibility in running is important, so make this a part of your regular exercise regimen. There are many resources available where you can learn more about stretching.

Many experts agree that stretching reduces muscle soreness after running and results in better athletic performance. Gentle stretching after a race or intense workout can also promote healing and lactic acid removal from the muscles. Stretching is most effective when performed several times each week; a minimum of one stretching session per week is sufficient to maintain flexibility. A predominance of coaches and runners believe in stretching before and after every workout.

According to my doctor, improper stretching is the second leading cause of running injuries for both runners who do not stretch very much and for runners who spend an inordinate amount of time stretching.

The bottom line is you should stretch before and after your runs, you should be gentle in your stretching, you should ensure your stretches are slow and you should hold the stretch. Bouncing into the stretch can cause more harm than good.

I often find I am able to stretch better after I've had a short warm-up run. This is especially true after a long run the day before. In these situations, I'll stretch for a few minutes and run for half or three-quarters of a mile. Then I'll stretch again. I find that my muscles respond better to stretching after they are warmed up.

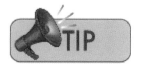 **Here's a Tip!** Do not stretch beyond the point where you begin to feel tightness in the muscle, do not push through muscle resistance, and never stretch to the point of discomfort or pain.

How to Stretch

Always remember to stretch slowly and hold the stretch for 30 to 40 seconds. You should try to build stretching into your regular schedule both before and after your daily run. A good program should include stretches for the calves, shins, hips, buttocks and thighs.

Here are some suggestions for stretches you can use.

Wall Pushup #1

This exercise will stretch your calve muscles. With your feet flat on the ground, and shoulder width apart, place your hands on a wall with your arms straight (you should be standing about three feet from the wall). Now, lean your hips toward the wall and bend your knees slightly. You should feel it in your calves.

Wall Pushup #2

Keep your feet in the same place and bend at the waist to a 90 degree position (hands on wall straight in front of you). Tuck your head down and look at your feet. Now, pull one foot forward with your knee slightly bent. Flex your toes up, feeling the stretch in the muscle below your calf. Repeat this exercise with your other leg.

Wall Pushup #3

Stay bent at the waist with your head tucked between your arms; pull your feet together in the same spot (about three feet from the wall). Now, flex both feet up while rocking back on your heels. Can you feel the stretch in your shoulders, lower back and hips? You should.

Hamstring Stretch

Now lie down on your back (on a firm surface like the ground outside or the floor inside). Bend your knee and pull your foot toward your bottom until it is flat on the ground. Now raise your other leg straight up in the air. Loop a T-shirt or towel over your raised foot (in the arch). With equal pressure gentle pull down as you push away with your foot. Pull and push only until you feel your muscles contracting. Repeat with opposite leg.

Heel to Buttock

Resume your position approximately three feet away from a wall. Place your left arm straight out with hand flat against the wall. Bend your right knee, and catch the bottom of your heel with your right hand behind your buttock. Pull your heel toward your buttock, get as close as you comfortably can. Repeat with opposite leg. This exercise stretches your quadriceps.

Groin Stretch

Sit on the ground with the soles of your feet together and pulled as close to your body as is comfortable. Place your elbows inside the crease at your knees and hold your ankles. Slowly push your knees toward the ground; stop when this becomes uncomfortable.

 **Here's a Tip!** I learned this one the hard way: Don't trip. I'm serious about this. In researching this book, I talked with three people who hurt themselves (one badly enough that she was not able to run her race) because they were in a runner's fog and fell. Pay attention out there.

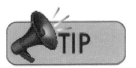 **Here's another Tip!** Your second marathon will be much easier and more pleasant than your first for one important reason: You'll know what to expect. This applies to your body, as well. When you're training for subsequent marathons, you will come to expect certain aches and pains at different stages of your training. Not only that, but you will get better at knowing what you can do to fix the problem.

Keep in mind that pain is an indicator that something is wrong with your body. Think of pain as a warning light on your car. If you have an unusual pain, think of it as a "check engine" light. Instead of ignoring it (like I often do with my car), go see your doctor.

10: THE NEXT SIXTEEN WEEKS

> "The woods are lovely dark and deep, but I have promises to keep,
> and miles to go before I sleep, and miles to go before I sleep."
>
> - Robert Frost, from the poem
> "Stopping by Woods on a Snowy Evening"

I am going to start this chapter with an admission: I can't run 26 miles, and I've never been able to. Yes, I said it. But before you call me a fraud, let me explain.

You see, when I run a marathon, I don't set out to cover 26 miles. That's too much to consider. I simply can't get my pea-brain around 26 miles. It's too much.

But, what I can do is think of the marathon as a series of shorter runs. So, when I think about running the marathon, or contemplate my longer runs, I break it down into smaller chunks that I *can* get my mind around. So, when I run a marathon, I don't think of it as 26 miles, I think of it as, roughly, four ten-kilometer runs, followed by a two mile warm down. I *can* do that...

Huh?, you ask.

In my long runs, such as my 18 or 20-mile training runs, I find it is helpful to start out thinking only of the first part of the run — usually a distance of about 10 kilometers, or just over 6 miles. I can usually run 6 miles in my sleep. Then, when I get to the 6-mile mark, I tell myself I am beginning another 6-mile run. Here again, even if I am worn out, I can run another 6 miles, no problem.

You see, running a marathon is never about running 26 miles in one shot. Instead, it is about running a smaller race multiple times.

I want you to keep that in mind as I discuss the training program in greater detail.

Introduction to the Training Program

A minute ago, I discussed the importance of breaking the race into smaller races. Now, I want use the same logic in regard to training.

Just the other night, my wife and I went to a party and the subject of running came up. At some point during the conversation, someone said, "I can run 3 miles at a time, but I could never run 26. That seems so *far*..." My response to this logic is always the same.

If you can run easily 3 miles, you *can* run 6 miles. That's a no-brainer. You can do it. Really. Then, after running 6 miles for a while and getting some level of comfort at that distance, you can run 12 miles. Yep, you can do it. If you run 12 comfortably — and yes, eventually it will become comfortable — you can run 16. If you can run 16 miles, you can run 20 and you can run a marathon.

"So," you ask, "if I can run 3 miles, does that mean that I can automatically run 26?"

Of course, you can't run 26 miles now. You have a lot of training to do. But if you can run 3 miles, you can eventually run 26.

My whole point is that your body can do it. The only thing keeping you from your marathon is your mind. I want you to keep that in your head as I discuss training in this chapter.

The Long Run

Before you begin this program, it is critical that you establish a running foundation. While you can get by with a little less, I think it is really important to be able to run, very comfortably, 6 miles at a time. You should also be running between 3 and 5 days per week, averaging between 15 and 25 miles per week. Ideally, you should have run one or more 5-10 kilometer races. Again, you can run a marathon with a less significant foundation, but believe me when I say it is far less fun and much riskier than if you have a solid running foundation.

The most important part of any marathon program is the weekly long run. As we move along in the program, you will notice we add miles every other week. During the interim weeks, our long runs will still be long, but we won't add miles.

The most important ingredient to marathon success is the long run; it mirrors the marathon itself. "Going long" is a hallowed weekend tradition that is despised and loved, feared and revered, bragged and complained about. First-time and casual marathoners should gradually increase the length of long runs and complete at least three runs of 18 to 20 miles prior to the marathon.

It is important for me to note that it is absolutely critical that you run every single long run. I mean it. You can't cheat on your long runs!

During the week, you will run shorter distances. The distance of these shorter runs will increase, as well, but less dramatically. As I mentioned before, it's a good idea to log your runs in your training log. Write down how you feel, what you ate before and after you ran, how well you recovered and, if you care (which I never do), your time.

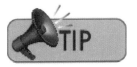 **Here's a Tip!** Take care in selecting your running routes. I like to find a route that is similar to the one I will run in the race, especially as it relates to hills. I also like a route that has drinking fountains or a place to stash water in bottles, and, ideally, at least one bathroom.

I've learned this lesson the hard way. A few years ago, during one of my longer runs, I started to have stomach pains. Fortunately, I was able to limp, quite literally, to a bathroom where I had a terrible case of diarrhea. Unfortunately, the park where the bathroom was located was my turnaround point, meaning I had to make it nine miles back to my car. I won't get into the sordid details of my bodily functions or my nine-mile walk back to my car. But I learned a valuable lesson about the importance of restrooms along your route.

The Leap of Faith

If you're like me, before you read this section, you probably skipped ahead to the middle of the training program and noticed we log some pretty long runs. You might be getting a little nervous (that's normal), and if you are a particularly astute reader, you noticed that while we run 20 miles three times, we never run more than 20 miles during our training. "So," you ask, "how can I run 26 miles when I have only trained for 20 miles?"

Ah, good question. First, I need to correct you. You *have* trained for 26 miles even though your longest run is only 20 miles. Training for a marathon is cumulative, based on your week of running. You will notice that during the weeks of running your longer run, you have weekly totals that reach 40 miles. Remember what I said earlier — a person who is able to comfortably run 3 miles is really able to run at least 6 miles. The same logic applies here. You can run 20 miles at one time comfortably, but during the race you will have the extra power, stamina and drive to run 26.

"So," you ask, "why don't we run 26 miles during our training runs?" That is another good question. That is exactly the same question I asked when I started training for my marathon. The bottom line is that running longer than 4 hours — and for most beginning marathoners, running 26 miles takes them longer than 4 hours, — results in extreme fatigue. Not only does it take a lot longer for your body to recover after a 4 hour run, but you are much more prone to injury.

Through the course of this book, I hope I've been able to gain some trust with you, friendly reader. So, I ask you to trust me that if you can complete the 20-mile runs I explain in this book, you can finish the marathon. I encourage you to talk with other marathon finishers about this. My guess is the vast majority of them never train past 20 miles.

Ground Rules

Before we get into the training program, it is important that we discuss some ground rules. I've already discussed one of the most important rules —the need to get your long runs in. There is another rule that is just as important: If something hurts, get it checked by a professional. By this point in the book, you probably think I'm a hypochondriac. I'm not. But I am experienced, and I'd hate for you to get hurt.

Running is hard work and, as we've discussed, it will hurt sometimes. You will also have some very stiff mornings. However, if you pay attention to your body, you will notice when something doesn't seem right. If it hurts, get it checked out.

The third ground rule I stress is that you re-read the sections on stretching and feeding the machine.

The fourth rule is also very important. I want you to take a few minutes during each of your runs and be proud of yourself. Acknowledge what you've accomplished this far. A year ago you wanted to run a marathon. Now, you are well on your way!

Base

In the weeks leading up to the beginning of your training, I want you to get used to running a program. This is the base I like to establish for myself. Mondays are always tough, so I generally don't run that day. I run short distances on Tuesday, Wednesday, and Thursday, and I take Friday off. I do my long run (six miles) for the week on Saturday, and then I have a nice, short recovery run the next day, Sunday, when I run three miles.

Monday	Tuesday	Wednesday	Thursday	Friday	Saturday	Sunday
off	4	3	4	off	6	3

Week One

During the first week of the program we will build ever so slightly on the base we have established. We'll follow the same schedule as our base with the exception of adding two miles to our long run on Saturday.

Monday	Tuesday	Wednesday	Thursday	Friday	Saturday	Sunday
off	4	3	4	off	8	3

Week Two

Our second week will be exactly the same as the first. Our goal is to get you used to the eight mile run.

Monday	Tuesday	Wednesday	Thursday	Friday	Saturday	Sunday
off	4	3	4	off	8	3

Week Three

You probably noticed the eight-miler in the second week was much easier than the first. Time to move on. The next two weeks will establish the routine we'll use for the rest of the program, adding miles in one week and then recovering with a shorter version of our "long run" the following week.

In week three, we are going to add two more miles to our Saturday run. Make sure you stretch and have plenty of water along your course. Are you getting blisters or chafing? If you are, talk with someone at your shoe store and change your gear. By this time, you are probably waking up a little stiff in the morning and you may be a little sore going up and down stairs. That, my friend, is pretty typical.

Monday	Tuesday	Wednesday	Thursday	Friday	Saturday	Sunday
off	4	3	4	off	10	3

Remember to have a nice slow stretch on Sunday. The goal of that run is simply for recovery. Don't kill yourself. Run nice and slowly!

Week Four

I love training weeks like week four. This is when we back off of our long run. After last week's ten-mile run, we're going to back off to eight miles. By now, your eight mile run will be relatively easy, but expect some soreness in your shorter weeks because of the extra mileage the previous week.

Are you proud of yourself? You should be.

How many people do you know who can go out and run ten miles? Not many.

You're doing great!

Monday	Tuesday	Wednesday	Thursday	Friday	Saturday	Sunday
off	4	3	4	off	8	3

Week Five

All right, we're back at it in week five. This is a big week. We're going to run 13 miles on Saturday, an addition of 3 miles to your longest run so far. This might seem like a big jump, but it really isn't as big as you think.

Remember those mind games I taught you earlier? Start using those now. Get fired up for this run — it's an important one.

Monday	Tuesday	Wednesday	Thursday	Friday	Saturday	Sunday
off	4	3	4	off	13	3

 **Here's a Tip!** That Sunday recovery run may be tough. If you find you are too sore to run that three-miler, go for a nice, fast walk or a relaxing bicycle ride. Don't kill yourself... Have a nice recovery. Don't forget to stretch.

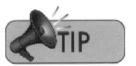 **Here's a Tip!** Start getting into a routine before your longer runs. I like to eat the same things before every long run, wear the same clothes for each long run, even say goodbye to my family in the same way before my long runs.

Week Six

If you are like me (and most people), you might be pretty stiff the first couple days after last week's long run It is critical that you rest a lot this week. No running and no working out on Monday at all. Get a nice slow run in on Tuesday, Wednesday and Thursday of this week. Don't overdo it.

Rest on Friday and have a nice and easy ten-miler on Saturday. You'll recover on Sunday.

Monday	Tuesday	Wednesday	Thursday	Friday	Saturday	Sunday
off	4	4	4	off	10	3

Here's a Tip! I tend to do my longer runs along the same route. That allows me to mentally prepare for longer runs, know where drinking fountains are located (or where I can stash water), and where I can get help or use a toilet, if needed. I know some fellow runners who like to run a different route each week, but not me. I like to know my course.

Week Seven

This week, we'll increase our mileage again. Don't worry if you're still a little sore at the beginning of the week. By the end of the week, you will feel much improved.

Are you eating well and sleeping well? You've probably noticed that your need for sleep and for good food has increased dramatically in the last few weeks. Give your body what it needs.

We'll run our normal four miles on Tuesday, Wednesday, and Thursday with a nice long fifteen-miler on Saturday, and an easy recovery run on Sunday.

Remember, don't do anything on Monday or Friday and try to stay off your feet as much as you can after your long run on Saturday.

Monday	Tuesday	Wednesday	Thursday	Friday	Saturday	Sunday
off	4	4	4	off	15	3

Week Eight

All right, we've been in the program for two months now. Here again, this week eight is another lower mileage week. You'll rest Monday and Friday, run a nice five-miler on Tuesday, followed by four-milers on Wednesday and Thursday. You'll run thirteen on Saturday followed by your regular three-mile recovery run on Sunday.

Monday	Tuesday	Wednesday	Thursday	Friday	Saturday	Sunday
off	5	4	4	off	13	3

Week Nine

This is a big week — we'll do our first eighteen-miler on Saturday. We'll run our regular fours on Tuesday, Wednesday, and Thursday. We'll stay off our feet Monday and Friday and have a nice slow recovery run on Sunday.

Monday	Tuesday	Wednesday	Thursday	Friday	Saturday	Sunday
off	4	4	4	off	18	3

Week Ten

Once again, this week you'll experience some stiffness and soreness, but your longer run will be shorter on Saturday. Make sure to stretch especially well before and after each of your runs.

Monday	Tuesday	Wednesday	Thursday	Friday	Saturday	Sunday
off	4	4	4	off	13	3

Week Eleven

As you are out on your long run, I want you to carve out some time to reflect on your new ability to run 20 miles. It's quite an accomplishment. I also want you to start thinking about your next challenge. In training for a marathon, you've taken on a huge challenge. You are well on your way to accomplishing it. Now, I want you to think about what is next. It might be a long bike race, climbing a mountain, sailing around the world, doing a triathlon, or writing a book. I don't care what it is; I just want you to start planning your next challenge now.

Monday	Tuesday	Wednesday	Thursday	Friday	Saturday	Sunday
off	4	4	4	off	20	3

Week Twelve

Nice and easy this week. You are going to be a little sore. Start your runs slowly and keep yourself well-hydrated.

Monday	Tuesday	Wednesday	Thursday	Friday	Saturday	Sunday
off	4	4	4	off	13	3

Week Thirteen

Here we go! You've got a longer run this week. Believe me, it will be easier than the first.

Monday	Tuesday	Wednesday	Thursday	Friday	Saturday	Sunday
off	4	4	4	off	20	3

Week Fourteen

All right! We're going to add one mile on Wednesday. Nice and easy this week. Don't forget to stretch.

Monday	Tuesday	Wednesday	Thursday	Friday	Saturday	Sunday
off	4	5	4	off	13	3

Week Fifteen

This is it—your last 20-mile run. Enjoy it; it's all much easier from here! Congratulate yourself.

Monday	Tuesday	Wednesday	Thursday	Friday	Saturday	Sunday
off	4	5	4	off	20	3

Week Sixteen

Once again, this week you'll experience some stiffness and soreness, but you'll have a shorter long run on Saturday. Make sure to stretch, especially well before and after each of your runs. It's probably hard to believe, but after your 15-miler on Saturday, you are done with your long runs.

Just one more week of hard running. Make it a good one, because after this, you are tapering.

Remember to imagine running the race when you run your long run. Drink what you will drink during the race, eat what you will eat during the race. Imagine yourself with a number on your chest actually running your race.

When you are done, raise your hands in the air in victory. You are done with the hardest part of your training. You've done it, and you should be very, very proud!

Monday	Tuesday	Wednesday	Thursday	Friday	Saturday	Sunday
off	4	4	4	off	15	3

11: THE TAPER

Aut viam inveniam aut faciam.

- Translation: I'll either find a way or make one.

Congratulations!

You've made it through your training runs and are tapering before your big race. Feels strange, doesn't it?

In this chapter, I'll discuss the last couple weeks before your marathon. I'm also going to provide you with some tips and offer some other advice. My most important job at this point in your training is to reassure you and let you know you are going to be fine. You are going to make it. We'll come back to this in just a second.

The Importance of Rest

The most important thing you should do during your taper period is to rest your body. Rest means no running beyond what is called for in the program. This also means no cross-training. Rest doesn't mean swapping swimming for running or going for a long bike ride every day. Rest means rest. Put your feet up. Relax. Catch up on your TV-watching. Rest!

If you missed a few runs during the last 16 weeks, want to lose a few more pounds or really want to work on a few more hills, or whatever it is, you need to know this. If you haven't lost the weight, run the hills or logged the miles, you should not try to do it now. The best thing you should do, and the only thing you should do, is rest. Am I clear?

But, Can I Do It?

By this time, because you've put in all these miles, your body wants you to keep running. You might even be longing to run, and you'll feel guilty about not running. Often at this stage in your preparation, a little self-doubt creeps into people's minds. The internal conversation goes something like this:

"Can I really run 26 miles? I only ran 20 miles three times... Am I ready? Won't all of this rest make me rusty? Am I going to be a complete failure?"

Let me tell you as forcefully as I can that, yes, you will make it. Your training has prepared you. You are ready.

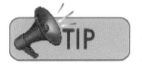 **Here's a Tip!** As you scale back on the distance and intensity of your workouts during your taper, you have to realize you aren't burning as many calories as you did prior to your taper. Remember those pounds you shed in the last several weeks? Be careful in selecting foods to eat during this time period so you don't gain them back. Select quality foods, rather than high-fat, low-nutrition junk.

The Last Weeks

Again, the goal of the taper in the last two weeks of our program is to rest, recuperate, and to mend our bodies before the race. That said, you can have some nice slow runs. Don't go over the suggested mileage! You're going to want to test your legs, but don't do it. Your main job now is to rest, so rest!

At this point, make sure you are reading ahead about the weeks and days before the race. You're probably nervous. That section will put your mind at ease.

Week Seventeen

Monday	Tuesday	Wednesday	Thursday	Friday	Saturday	Sunday
off	5	4	off	4	4	3

Week Eighteen

Monday	Tuesday	Wednesday	Thursday	Friday	Saturday	Sunday
off	4	4	off	2	4	Race!

12: LEADING UP TO THE RACE

> *"We are different, in essence, from other men. If you want to win something,*
> *run 100 meters. If you want to experience something, run a <u>marathon</u>."*
>
> - Emil Zatopek

Can you believe it's almost race time? Here you are, just a few weeks from completing your marathon mission. How do you feel? Are you tired? Are you nervous?

All of these feelings are very normal. In this section, I am going to provide some advice in those areas to help you as you lead up to the race...

Two Weeks Before:

There are several things we need to do at this stage of the game. Let's go over them.

Visualize your Success

While you're relaxing, I encourage you to visualize the race. In your mind, envision yourself finishing. Imagine yourself crossing the finish line. How will you feel? What will it look like? Spend some time every day visualizing your success.

Make sure you are eating well. Your body is repairing and replenishing itself. Give it what it needs.

Prepare your Supporters

If you've done your job talking about the marathon, then you probably have some people who want to come out and cheer you on. This is both a blessing and a curse. You want people to support you, but in some cases, managing your supporters is a chore itself.

Do yourself a favor and ask a spouse or close friend to be the main contact for your supporters — designate him or her to be your support coordinator. That way, you can worry about more pressing issues, like running a marathon.

Encourage your support coordinator to place people strategically along the course. You will want people at mile 20, but don't put all of your supporters at the end of the race. If you have a lot of people, scatter groups of people every three, five or seven miles.

 **Here's a Tip!** Know where to expect your supporters, but don't worry if you miss them. Also, don't slow down or stop and prepare to say a few words of thanks as you run by. Also, watch other people as their friends and family cheer for them as they run by.

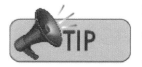

Here's another Tip! Your friends and family will think they are doing you a favor by offering you food and drink. Don't take it. If you have done a good job selecting your marathon, water and other fluids should not be a problem. Don't introduce new food at this late stage. You'd be asking for problems.

Here's another Tip! Will your mother or your kids be in the crowd? Moms and little kids should be along the course, but, if you can, let them know you are feeling good—smile and wave as you're running by. My experience with moms and kids suggests they both want to know you are okay. I always try to slow down enough to give my kids a high-five, my wife a sweaty hug and my mom a reassuring thumbs-up.

Ready Your Gear

By now, you should have tested all of your running clothes in your long runs and have broken-in, race-ready gear. During your taper, wear that gear for every run.

Get your running fuel together and your sports drinks and gels. If you are going to carry gels while you run, buy several extra.

Most larger marathons provide clear plastic bags with ties that you bring to the starting area. Before the race, you can put warm-ups, extra food and other items that you want at the start-line and will want again at the finish-line in the bag. These are things you don't want to wear or carry. Most of the time, the bag has a number on a sticker which corresponds with a truck or van number. Prior to the start of the race, check your bag and you can pick it up at the finish. I like to check my bag early. This gives me one less thing to worry about.

The worst thing you can do at the beginning of the race is to allow yourself to get cold. To avoid getting cold, I bring an old pair of sweats, two trash bags, an old hat and gloves to the start. I intend to throw all of it away at the beginning of the race, so I don't have to worry about checking it in.

Some marathons, including the New York City Marathon, make this very easy; they have specific drop-off points at the beginning of the race for you to throw out your old clothes. The organizers of the marathon donate all the clothes to the needy.

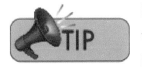 **Here's a Tip!** Take off your sweat pants prior to lining up for the race. Especially in the larger races, the line of runners, even before the marathon begins, tends to move slowly toward the line. This means it's hard to remove a pair of pants after you've lined up. In most cases, your legs won't get as cold as your upper body, so ditch the pants and keep a loose-fitting sweatshirt that you can easily remove while you are running. I also like to wear a stocking hat for the first mile. I don't know if it really helps keep me warm or if it just makes me feel like Rocky. Either way, it works for me.

One Week Before:

I was a wreck one week before my first marathon. I was hungry, tired (but not sleeping well), and had a constant knot in my stomach. I also couldn't understand why I wasn't training. It seemed like the more I rested, the more I felt like I should be running.

The week before my second marathon was much better. I knew I would be able to run the race. I was able to calm down, enjoy my rest and look forward to the marathon. As I said before, you've earned your down-time. Enjoy it.

Listen, you are going to be excited. You are going to be nervous. The best thing you can do this week is to know you are going to have a great marathon. I promise. Stay off your feet as much as you can. Go to the movies or watch movies at home. Call some old friends and catch up. Eat well and keep yourself hydrated. Stay busy, but stay relaxed.

The Day Before the Race:

How are you doing? Feeling very nervous, having some self-doubt and wondering if this whole "marathon thing" is a good idea is completely normal. Again, you are fine. Here are some thoughts.

Do what you can to stay off your feet today. Don't run and try to walk as little as possible. Take a nap, watch TV, eat good carbohydrates and drink lots of good fluids. Rest, relax and enjoy life.

In terms of nutrition, be sure to eat carbohydrate products that have been "tried and proven" during your training period. Keep pasta sauces simple, avoiding high fat varieties (e.g., alfredo, pesto, etc.).

Avoid eating lots of salad items and vegetables (roughage), because these may prove to be troublesome on race day as they may cause digestive problems. Stick to water during the evening meal. Because coffee and tea contain caffeine, these products may make it difficult for you to fall asleep easily. Caffeine (along with alcoholic beverages) is a diuretic which can lead to dehydration.

I'd encourage you to pick up your number and other race material as soon as you can. Then, you can make sure everything is ready to go. Pin your number on your shirt and get all of your gear ready. If the marathon uses a "chip" to record times, lace it into your shoes as per the instructions.

If possible, I strongly recommend you visit the finish line today. More than likely the organizers of the race are setting up the finish area. Go see it. If possible, spend some time looking at the finish line. Visualize yourself in the race running across the line.

Set your running clothes out, along with several layers that will keep you warm at the start line. I like to bring along a garbage bag that can be used as a raincoat if it's raining or I need a dry place to sit in the morning dew.

Go to bed early and set two alarm clocks. Smile, you are almost there.

The Morning of the Race

I like to get to the start line right away in the morning, so I tend to get up early on race day. Put on your clothes and have a good breakfast with an extra portion of carbohydrates. Have an extra glass of water along with some Gatorade or another sports drink. Here again, this is not the day to try something new. If you eat oatmeal every morning for breakfast, eat oatmeal today.

I like to write little words of encouragement on the palm of my hand, some place where no one will see. For my last marathon I wrote, "I will either find a way or make one."

Have a few minutes of alone-time with a spouse and talk over the race. I find that this is a great time to give a few words of thanks. If you are a spiritual person, give a few words of thanks to your maker. You are going to have one of the greatest days of your life.

Pre-Race

The best advice anyone can give you right before your marathon is to enjoy it. You will be nervous. You wouldn't be human if you weren't nervous. Have some water and something to eat between two hours and thirty minutes before the start. Again, stay off your feet and stay warm. Relax. You are almost there.

13: THE RACE

"We can't all be heroes because someone has to sit on the curb and clap as they go by."

- Will Rogers

Your Race: The First Six Miles

Run your race in exactly the same way you ran your long training runs. Find your rhythm and pace. You are going to be excited, so you will have to work to slow yourself down.

I like to run alongside or right behind two runners who are running next to each other and are running the same pace as me. I figure they are more likely to run a constant pace than a single person. If they are too fast or too slow, I pick someone else.

Talk to yourself to calm yourself down. Remind yourself that you are making good on your promise to yourself. Enjoy the crowds. Do you hear them cheering? They are cheering for you. This is your day.

Don't worry about your time — enjoy the run. Stay controlled when you run, stay loose and remember to move stretch your upper body every now and then and move your toes around.

Do not pass up any fluid station. While it's okay to drink only water in the early miles, runners must consume sports beverages no later than after 90 minutes of running (and earlier if possible). Find out what works best for you in long practice runs.

Water is usually offered at the first tables at an aid station, with sports beverages served near the end of the station. Squeeze the top of the cup into a "v" shape to create a smooth delivery of fluid directly into your mouth if you choose to run and drink through the aid stations. If necessary, walk through the aid stations to be sure you are able to consume the entire contents of the cup. If you decide to stop and drink, please get out of the way of other runners.

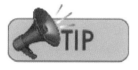 **Here's a Tip!** Remember to be careful of crushed drinking cups—they get slippery in the roadway—also watch out for discarded clothing.

Your Race: The Second Six Miles

Are you still hydrated?

Are you running too fast?

By the second six miles, you should have settled into your pace. You will probably be amazed at how quickly those first six miles went. Stay loose and stay focused.

Your Race: The Third Six Miles

At this point, you are probably amazed at how strong you feel. The most important thing you can do is stay hydrated, stay focused and stay loose. Stick with your game plan. Enjoy the ride!

Your Race: The Fourth Six Miles

At this point you've run 18 miles. Some people think this is the hardest part of the race, but not me — this is my favorite part of the race. You should continue to stay focused (don't let your mind drift), and keep the fluids coming. Stay loose and keep your good form.

During this part of the race, I like to look ahead at the people on the side of the course. I give little kids high-fives and chat it up with my fellow runners. I actually had a great conversation with a man from France at mile eighteen. That was fun.

One of my most vivid memories came during my very first marathon when, at mile twenty as we ran into the Bronx during the New York City Marathon, I ran next to a man who ran on prosthetic legs. As we ran together, we both passed an older man who was in a wheelchair, as he pulled himself up and over a bridge with one leg.

As I ran, tears streamed down my face — I can't tell you how proud I was to run with those guys.

Your Race: The Last Two Miles

This is what it is all about, my friend. The last two miles are your victory lap. You have done the hard work and now your job is to simply enjoy the crowd, enjoy the company of your fellow runners and start enjoying your accomplishment.

I cherish the memories of the last two miles of my marathons. By this time, I know I am going to finish. I remind myself how proud I am and how proud others are of me. Make sure you keep your fluids up and have a gel if you planned to have one.

Take it all in... You are almost there. By the way, I have always cried at some point during the last two miles of my marathons. By this point, I am so elated, so proud and just so happy that I always shed more than a few tears. The marathon is immensely personal and, in the last two miles, you will see lots of people crying with joy.

Your Race: YOU DID IT!

Congratulations! You did it! You set a goal and ran your first marathon!

The most important thing you can do post-marathon is to keep walking. Walk and walk and walk some more. You will want to sit down, but don't do it. Drink some water and if your stomach is up to it, have a bagel.

By this time, you should have the foil blanket draped around your shoulders and a finisher's medal around your neck. Keep that blanket on for a while, you might be hot now, but you will cool down fast. Keep walking, keep drinking and stay warm. That's all you need to do.

If you're dizzy, have blisters or another injury, or just don't feel right, get some help right away. Don't be a hero — tell a volunteer you need some help.

Keep walking. Pick up your bag, meet your friends and family, and walk some more. Make sure you stretch as you walk, put some sugar back into your body and whatever you do, don't lay down.

Make sure you get some good food back into your stomach. Your body will crave carbohydrates, but make sure you have some protein and electrolytes. At this point, a sports drink is a better option than water. Grab some fruit and eat and drink slowly.

If you are in a larger marathon, take a nice long walk, more than a mile, back to your hotel or car. After showering, put some dry clothes on and try to stay off your feet for a while.

If you have blisters, treat them after your shower and make sure you keep them clean and bandaged. I use Band-Aid Advanced Healing bandages and New Skin Liquid Bandage.

It is important that you do some walking. The post-marathon party is a great way to celebrate your accomplishment, just don't do too much dancing.

I made the mistake a few years ago, after running the New York City Marathon, of following my family around New York City all night, including taking a trip to the giant Toys 'R Us store in Times Square. Finally, I had to just sit down on the floor — my legs were dead. Bad idea.

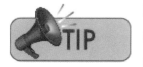

Here's a Tip! I'm not one to give parental advice, but I do want to encourage you to spend some alone time with your kids after the marathon. Again, you'll want to show them that you're fine after the race, but also thank them for their support and for cheering for you. Use your accomplishment as an opportunity to talk more about the importance of setting and reaching goals.

14: YOU DID IT! NOW WHAT?

"I have met my hero, and he is me."

- George Sheehan

After their first marathons, most runners do one of two things, both of which are bad. A lot of people start running right away. They feel so good after their marathon that they lace up their shoes a few days after their race and resume training.

It's important to realize that running 26 miles is a lot more taxing on your body that running 20 miles. Your body needs some time to heal. There is a lot of advice out there about when you should start running again...

You should view the next four to six weeks as a reverse taper. Not running for the first week will help you more than light running. Rest. The next week, you'll do some 20 to 30-minute runs and build it back up over the subsequent weeks. Eat healthy. A high carbohydrate diet in the first few days will help replenish your depleted carb storage system, and protein will help to rebuild damaged muscle tissue. Soups, juices, breads and a lot of healthy food will probably taste great, too. Get lots of sleep, take some easy walks, and you'll be ready to run again in no time. Remember the basic recovery process takes about a month. During this time, you'll have to continue to rest, run easy, avoid speed work, and keep your carbohydrate load high.

If you performed well in one marathon, be careful not to run and race too soon afterward because you are at a high risk for injury during the next six to eight weeks. Running another marathon, a fast 10K or 10-miler, or deciding to do another 20-mile training run between marathons that are spaced too close together could be enough to cause a lingering injury.

The rule of one day of recovery for each mile raced, or perhaps one day for each kilometer raced for master runners and novices, is a rule to keep in mind. Make sure you take the time to properly recover. If you are having serious pain, more than the usual post-marathon aches and pains, you should visit a sports medicine specialist. Otherwise, follow the advice in this article to try to prevent injury and allow for recovery.

Run Again? Are you Crazy?

A few weeks after my first marathon, I told some friends that my first marathon would be my last. It wasn't that it was a bad experience — it was one of the best in my life. I was simply tired ... of running.

Of course, I started running again when I felt like it, but I had a few months where I didn't feel like doing much of any kind of exercise. I was burnt out. This, I have learned, is pretty typical. My rule of thumb is that if you don't feel like doing it, don't do it.

However, I do encourage you to do something physical. You've probably lost a lot of weight and are in the best shape of your life. Just as we discussed earlier, now is the time to take on another challenge. It's also time to continue the good habits you developed. If you don't want to run for a while, try swimming.

Want to do something with your kids? Take them mountain biking. Want a fun weekend in the snow? Take up cross country skiing. Like the old Nike slogan says,

"Just Do It."

Final Thoughts

When I started writing this book, I wanted to do more than just tell people how to run a marathon. I wanted to take the mystery out of the marathon. I also wanted to use the marathon to empower the reader, just as I have been empowered by my running marathons.

I truly believe it is impossible to be the same person after running a marathon that you were before. At the very least, you've shown yourself and anyone else paying attention that you can set and achieve goals.

Through the course of your training, you and I have been on what I hope has been a wonderful journey. If I've accomplished anything with this book, I hope you have been inspired to make your dreams a reality—whatever those dreams are. I hope you learned that if you set your mind to it, you can accomplish your marathon mission. Most of all, I hope you are empowered and that you empower others around you to take chances, follow dreams and take on their own marathon missions.

See you at the finish line.

Your friend,

Joe Donovan

15: ADDITIONAL RESOURCES

> *"I decided to go for a little run."*
>
> - Forest Gump

Running Clubs: Some of the best resources available come from other runners. Talk to other runners and find a local running club. Weekly club runs often break up your training routine and can be a great way to meet new, like-minded people.

MapMyRun.com: This is a terrific website that allows you to plan your runs. Have lots of different running routes? You can store them on your account and use them again and again. This is a great resource.

Runner's Word: I find a lot of inspiration from Runner's World Magazine and a lot of useful information from the training sections. Definitely recommended.

Would you like to contribute other ideas for this section? E-mail us at:

ideas@marathonmethod.com.

ACKNOWLEDGEMENTS

Writing this book gave me the opportunity to think about and thank all those who helped me run my first marathon, and whose constant support has allowed me to accomplish other goals, including writing this book.

My parents, Joan and Jerry Donovan, taught me the importance of competing, not to win, but in learning how to win and lose. These are lessons I am proud to pass along to my children.

My older brothers, Steve and Dan, have long been my idols, and I look up to them now as much as I ever have, if not more.

My mother-in-law, Lonna Taylor, has been to all of my marathons and is a constant source of support for me, Leah, and our children.

My kids, Layne, Neave and Tighe, are my cheering section. Their chants of "Go, Dad, Go!" help me put one foot in front of the other, mile after mile after mile.

Finally, this book is dedicated to my wife, Leah, whose calm reassurance and unwavering confidence in me and my abilities has kept me looking for challenges and following my dreams. I love you more than you can know.

ABOUT THE AUTHOR

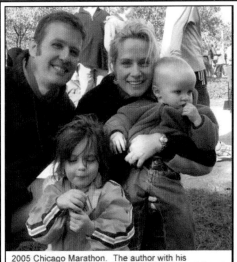

2005 Chicago Marathon. The author with his daughters Layne (blue jacket and finishers' medal) and Neave (pink jacket), son Tighe (in utero) and the love of his life, Leah.

Joe Donovan is a business owner, father, husband, runner and cyclist. Since running his first marathon in 1999, Joe has run three additional marathons and has completed a triathlon and several bicycle races. He is currently training for a long distance mountain bike race and maintains the website, MarathonMethod.com.

Joe and his family live in Wisconsin.

Joe can be reached at joe@marathonmethod.com.

Published by Julian John Publishing,
a division of the Donovan Group Holdings LLC.

JULIANJOHN

7445856R0

Made in the USA
Lexington, KY
22 November 2010